Essential Oils For Beginners

Best Guide To Get Started With Aromatherapy and Organic Recipes With Essential Oils

Table of Content:

Introduction 4

Chapter 1 – Essential Oil Recipes For Stress and Anxiety 7

Chapter 2 – Essential Oil Recipes for Relaxation 13

Chapter 3 – Essential Oil Recipes For Healing 19

Chapter 4 – Essential Oil Recipes for Sleep ... 23

Chapter 5 – Essential Oil Recipes for Hair Growth 31

Chapter 6 – Essential Oil for Cancer and Other Diseases 35

Conclusion 44

Introduction

Since the ancient times it is known that essential oils are very beneficial to our overall health. Before we experienced the advancement of modern medicine, essential oils are already present because they are already been used by our forefathers in several purposes.

When it comes to ingredients you will not find any flaws on them because they are completely all-natural or in other words they are a product of different herbs that are combined together to become worthy of your attention.

Before I was really skeptical about it because I thought how come will an essential oil cure such ailments? I tried several ways on how to cure my asthma but did not find any answer even on the medicines that the doctor is giving me that's why, what I did is to go for alternative medicines. This is where I came across the so-called essential oils, I did not knew that it will take a lot of effect on my overall health in a positive way.

To tell you frankly, my problem with my asthma has been completely resolved. I was really shocked with the results because I did not expect that a natural way of healing will suffice the need to cure my chronic condition.

Within a few days, my chronic condition got healed which made me feel happy because I felt a lot of relief. This is the primary reason why I decided to create a book that tackles the different essential oils that you can utilize to help you with your dilemmas.

I personally tried these recipes and they are really effective that's why you are in good hands because you have the peace of mind that it will work and you do not need to experiment anymore because I experimented them and tried it myself.

So by imparting these recipes with you, I have this joy of sharing and at the same time helping you to become overall well. Do not worry because all of the essential oils that we will tackle here are completely safe to use. And as a matter of fact I did not experience any allergic reactions from them.

As you will notice in the following chapters there are essential oils that are repeated because they have more than one use. It is the fact because herbal medicines are proven to target more than one condition.

Do not worry because it does not mean that if you are using an essential oil it tells that you have sickness because essential oils can be used for various purposes which we will discuss further in this book. So brace yourselves as we dive deeper into the different essential oils and their corresponding uses.

Chapter 1 – Essential Oil Recipes For Stress and Anxiety

Stress is prevalent nowadays and became a part of our day to day existence here on the planet. It is an immediate action of our body to combat the threats that we have either negative or not. The dilemma happens when stress stays longer than usual, which results in depression and other types of mental illnesses.

The Role of Essential Oils in Relieving Stress

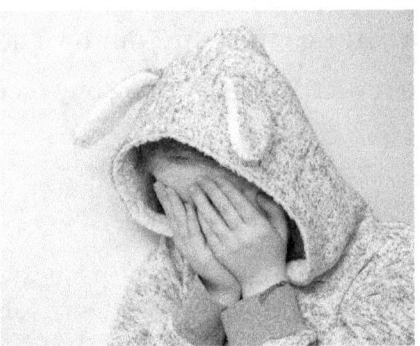

Stress can originate from different scenarios that we experience in our lives. We are lucky that there are natural techniques to support you in recovering from stress so that it will not elevate into something worse.

Thankfully, the concept of essential oils is invented because of them a lot of problems can now be cured naturally without any hassles.

They are very effective in releasing stress aside from that they can also enhance our performance and energy on everything that we do. Scientific research with essential oils particularly citrus has shown a significant improvement in their mental state.

Here are some examples of essential oil recipes that you can do at the comforts of your own home to relieve stress without undergoing any medical procedure.

Lavender and Clary Sage Blend

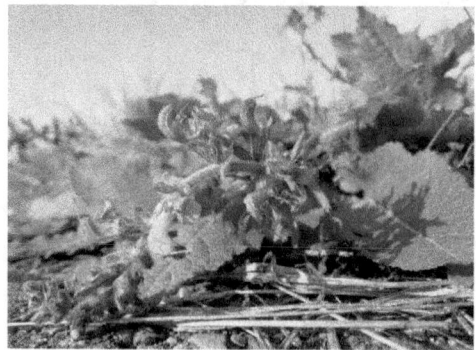

There are instances that stress can lead to sleep deprivation. The proceeding combinations of essential oils will aid you in sleeping rapidly which will result in lessening of stress in your life.

Lemon oil (5 drops)

Clary Sage (8 drops)

Lavender oil (5 drops)

Almond oil (2 drops)

Massage the combination of those essential oils among your hands and breathe in the aroma. Then continue doing it at the back of your neck and downwards. You can sense the pressure being released out of your body.

Sandal Wood Essential Oil Blend Recipe

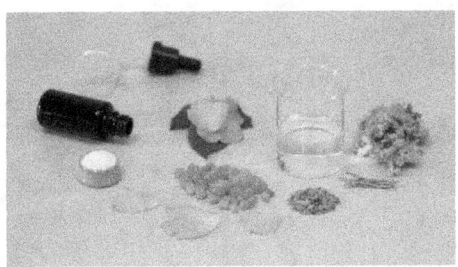

Put 5 drops of vetiver and 5 drops of sandalwood to the water that you will be used in taking a bath and then unwind while gasping the aroma.

Ylang-Ylang and Valerian Essential Oil Blend Recipe

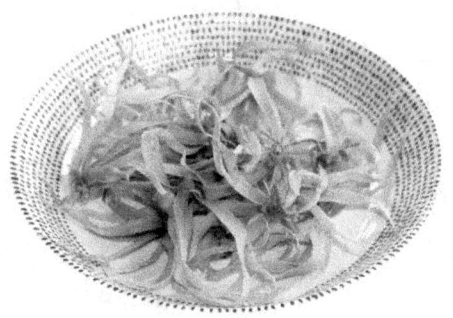

Mix 3 drops of valerian essential oil with 5 drops of ylang-ylang. Put it to you're the water that you will be using when you are going to take a bath.

Lavender and Peppermint Essential Oil Blend Recipe

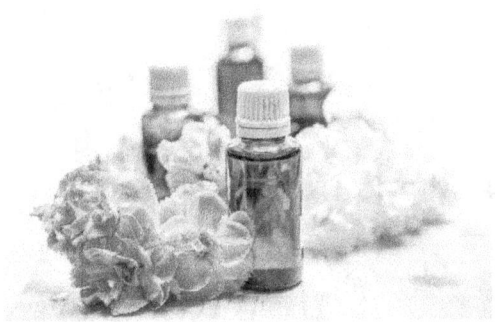

Mix 5 drops of lavender with 3 drops of peppermint essential oil or place it in a diffuser or water that you use when taking a bath.

Lavender and Chamomile Essential Oil Blend Recipe

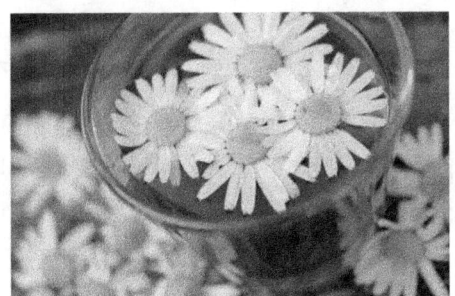

This recipe is good for any kinds of stress just mix 5 drops of lavender essential oil with 4 drops of chamomile oil. Just inhale it whenever you want to or put it on the water that you use in taking a bath.

Essential Oil Blend Recipes for Anxiety

Mix the succeeding essential oils:

Chamomile (16 drops)

Bergamot (2 drops)

Lavender (7 drops)

Geranium (7 drops)

Citrus (8 drops)

How to do it?

Place 2 tbsp of course sea salt in a container.

Place the blends inside it.

Blend them completely and cover it afterward.

Inhale this recipe three times up to 6 times a day to help you resolve your migraine problems.

Chapter 2 – Essential Oil Recipes for Relaxation

There are times when we feel that we are exhausted from the everyday work that we do because of that our energies are drained throughout our body. This is the primary reasons why we look for ways on how to rejuvenate ourselves to bring back the energy loss from the tasks that we do. One way is through the use of essential oils because it is all natural and very effective on its purpose.

Throughout the years a lot of essential oil blend recipes are created to help us relax and soothe our minds for us to function much better whenever needed. Here are some of the recipes that you can make at the comforts of your own home.

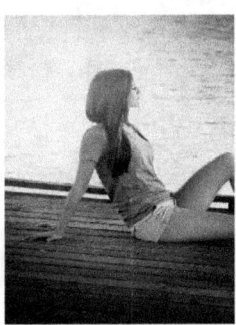

Lavender and Chamomile Blend

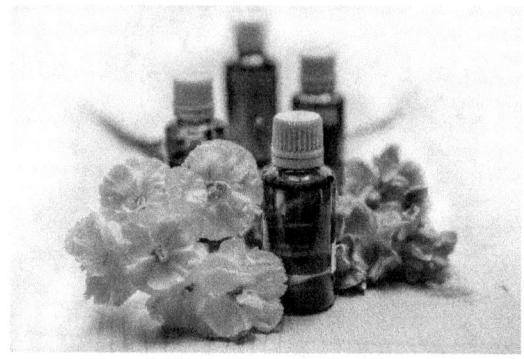

Lavender is popular among the most mainstream and flexible essential oils because it has fragrant healing benefits that can improve your general wellbeing. Since it is it can be used to beautify our skin, heal certain diseases, and restore our health.

What's more? it is also good for the development and maintenance of our brain. Lavender effects the mind similar to what medicines do. When you blend it with chamomile - another essential oil that quiets the nerves - the unwinding boosting properties are much tougher. Chamomile has been demonstrated to battle nervousness and wretchedness.

Lavender and Bergamot

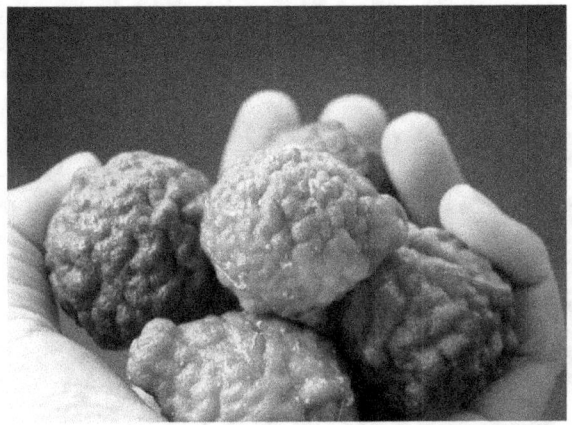

In the event that you are attempting to loosen up because of an unpleasant day, you need fragrant healing that will bring you back on track. In the event that you already have some lavender, add bergamot to add more zen to the recipe.

Studies show different fragrance based treatment benefits; bergamot catches the enormous three for advancing mental unwinding, lessening your circulatory strain, pulse, and feeling of anxiety. It likewise mitigates physical agony that can meddle with genuine feelings of serenity.

Lavender, Bergamot, Frankincense, and Cedarwood

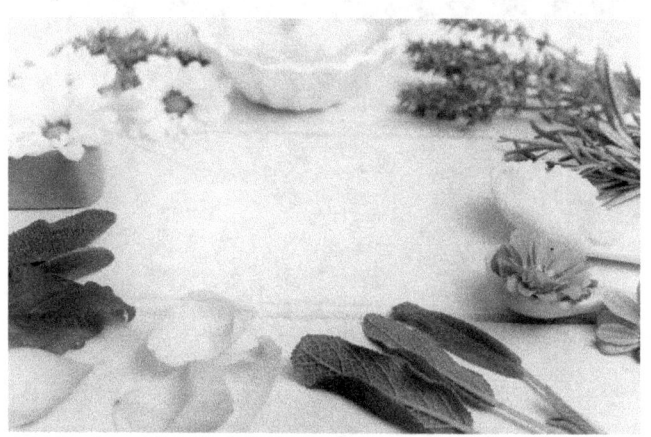

Its been logically demonstrated that, with fragrance-based treatment, you don't need to compromise your magnificence rest. As indicated by different medical professionals, an amazing tranquilizer includes blending bergamot, lavender, frankincense, and cedarwood in a jug.

You can even test these oils independently to check whether they help balance your sleep deprivation.

Lemon and Eucalyptus

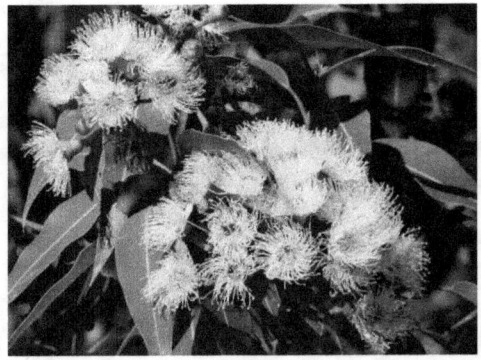

The failure to unwind can prompt interminable pressure and unstable overall health. Fortunately, the blend of lemon and eucalyptus can help mitigate your cold and sinus disease. Lemon is a phenomenal decongestant with antiviral properties, while eucalyptus encourages breathing through a stuffy nose.

Steaming your face with a towel set over your head and bowl of boiling water is unwinding in itself. Include a couple of drops of these oils for a quieting knowledge that will soothe a lot of your dilemmas regarding your health.

Frankincense, Cedarwood, and Chamomile

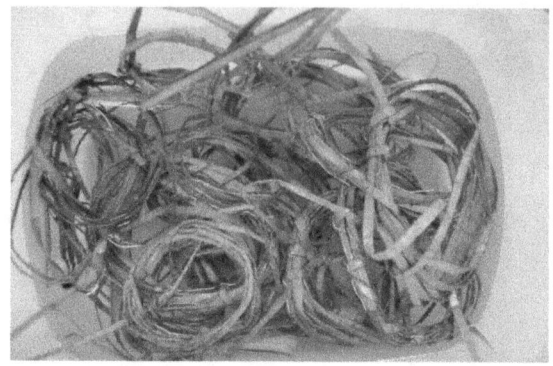

When you can't release it, attempt frankincense.
This essential oil has been utilized for a
considerable length of time to help individuals
ponder. At the point when matched with cedarwood
and chamomile, it is significantly increasingly
strong in calming the brain.

Chapter 3 – Essential Oil Recipes For Healing

Believe it or not, the best essential oils that we know today are the latest in plant-based treatments. To be reasonable, ancient people practiced various distillation strategies, however, the essential oils that were removed hundreds of years prior were really different from are accessible to us today.

Nevertheless, they all contained essential oils and extremely successful at avoiding and any unforeseen sickness.

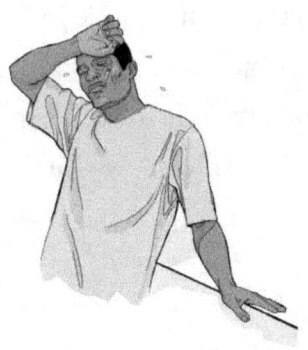

It is said that ancient people were delighted in by those in old Cyprus, Egypt and Pompeii who originally utilized herbs with refining strategies going back 3,500 B.C. This insight cruised over the Mediterranean and clearly achieved Hippocrates, who used fragrance based treatment to their immune systems a couple of hundreds of years before the happening to Christ.

As technology exchanged force to be reckoned with, the method of utilizing the best essential oils for healing from Greece went to Rome, who preferred fragrant healing and aromas.

Master the art of blending essential oils at the comforts of your own home! To help you achieve your wellbeing objectives with fundamental oils if it's not too much trouble make certain to set aside the effort to gain proficiency with the basics of aroma based treatment.

The best essential oils for healing are composed of various particles that each convey various impacts on the body.

Here is the rundown of the best essential oils to use for healing

Clove (Eugenia Caryophyllata)

Clove essential oil is generally utilized as a disinfectant for infections mostly the oral ones and to wipe out a wide range of organisms to keep ailment under control. It is known to combat a lot of bacteria such as E. coli and furthermore applied significant power over Staph aureus and Pseudomonas aeruginosa which are two microscopic organisms that are the main causes of pneumonia and skin contaminations.

Eucalyptus Globulus

This essential oil is used mostly by the Aborigines for most ailments in their tribe, eucalyptus is an effective antibacterial, antispasmodic, and antiviral oil. Like clove basic oil, eucalyptus basic oil has a significant effect over Staph contaminations. Did you know that when Staph aureus comes into contact with eucalyptus oil, the dangerous bacteria have totally lost control within a span of 15 minutes!

Frankincense

This essential oil has been utilized with much success in treating issues identified with bodily functions, immune system, oral wellbeing, respiratory concerns, and stress.

Lavender

Know for its alleviating and calming properties, lavender is great for quickening the recuperating time for wounds, stings, and various type of injuries. It is loaded with cancer prevention properties. It is also assessed for its capacity to treat diabetes and anxiety in rodents.

Lemon

Different citrus fundamental oils are broadly used to have healthy nodes, to revive slow, dull skin and as a bug repellent.

Chapter 4 – Essential Oil Recipes for Sleep

Diffusing essential oils for a good rest is one of the main things that got me interested in the world of essential oils.

Like most of us, I used to wake up 1 to 2 times each night. I'd hear the pooch strolling around, or my partner would turn over, or my psyche would race with every one of the things I needed to do the following day. I just couldn't appear to get the rest I desire. I was constantly worn out the next day because I did not get the sleeping hours that I need.

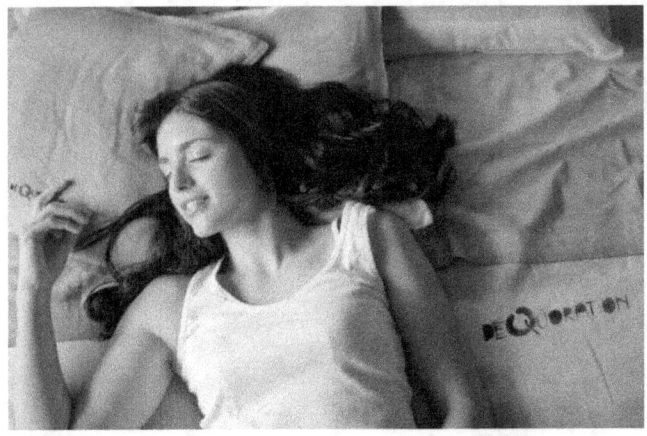

So this is when I try to experiment in using essential oils. I put 4 to 6 drops of lavender basic oil in a diffuser on the surface of my bed. Turned the diffuser on. Lie into my bed and floated off to rest.

Next thing I realized that it relieved the symptoms that I am experiencing before. I had rested straight during that time for an entire 9 hours "In any case, how could this be?" I thought it was just a coincidence.

So I attempted it again the following night. I topped off my diffuser with faucet water, and once more, I put a couple of drops of lavender essential oil in my diffuser. I transformed it on and went straight into my bed. Once more, I slept soundly as the night progressed, not awakening until I regained my consciousness back at 6:00.

There are many fundamental oils that help the psyche and body unwind

My preferred essential oils that help an incredible night's rest are lavender, cedarwood, vetiver, marjoram, frankincense, bergamot, sandalwood, Roman chamomile, patchouli, and orange.

Lavender

It is generally utilized for its calming properties. It facilitates pressure and initiates unwinding.

Cedarwood

The warm and woody fragrance that is both establishing and quieting, advancing an incredible night's rest

Vetiver

This grass has a rich, fascinating smell that is really great for manipulating your moods.

Marjoram

It has a warm fragrance that quiets and lets you diminish pressure and other types of anxiousness.

Roman Chamomile

It has a sweet botanical fragrance is quieting and alleviating to the brain and body, making it a standout amongst the frequently utilized essential oils for rest

Wild Orange

It's sweet citrus fragrance and, similar to bergamot, wild orange is an adaptogen that can be empowering or calming, contingent upon what your body needs

Patchouli

The musky aroma is establishing and great for managing your feelings

Hawaiian Sandalwood

It has a rich, sweet and woody fragrance imparts quiet and unwinding. It's alleviating fragrance decreases pressure, advances enthusiastic prosperity, and has a thoughtful impact.

Recipe # 1

Lavender essential oil (2 drops)

Cedarwood essential oil (2 drops)

Recipe #2

Bergamot essential oil (4 drops)

Lavender essential oil (5 drops)

Recipe #3

Lavender essential oil (2 drops)

Wild orange essential oil (2 drops)

Recipe #4

Lavender essential oil (3 drops)

Vetiver essential oil (3 drops)

Marjoram essential oil (3 drops)

Recipe #5

Roman chamomile essential oil (4 drops)

Bergamot essential oil (3 drops)

Frankincense essential oil (3 drops)

Recipe #6

Grounding blend essential oil (4 drops)

Lavender essential oil (3 drops)

Roman chamomile essential oil (3 drops)

Recipe #7

Lavender essential oil (3 drops)

Roman chamomile essential oil (3 drops)

Marjoram essential oil (3 drops)

Recipe #8

Patchouli essential oil (3 drops)

Wild orange essential oil (2 drops)

Frankincense essential oil (3 drops)

Recipe #9

Vetiver essential oil (4 drops)

Lavender essential oil (4 drops)

Frankincense essential oil (3 drops)

Recipe #10

Lavender essential oil (4 drops)

Vetiver essential oil (4 drops)

Recipe #11

Vetiver essential oil (4 drops)

Calming blend essential oil (4 drops)

Recipe #12

3 drops patchouli essential oil

3 drops sandalwood essential oil

Chapter 5 – Essential Oil Recipes for Hair Growth

Another advantage of essential oils have is its capacity to enhance our hair. Various oils can do everything from helping the hair to sparkle and to become stronger.

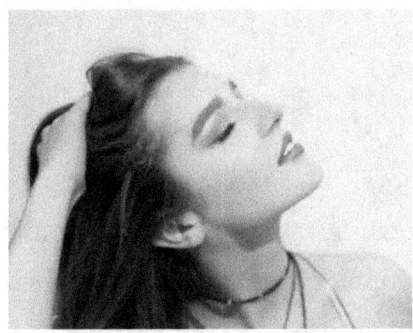

Here are the most effective essential oils for your hair:

Lavender

It can accelerate hair development. Realizing that lavender oil has properties that can create the development of cells and lessen pressure, scientists on one creature examine found that this oil had the option to produce quicker hair development in mice.

It also has antimicrobial and antibacterial properties, which can improve scalp wellbeing. Blend a few drops of lavender oil into 3 tablespoons of bearer oil, similar to olive oil or softened coconut oil, and apply it generously to your scalp. Let it sit for 10 minutes before washing it out and shampooing as you typically would. You can do this a few times each week.

Peppermint

Peppermint oil can cause a cool, shivering inclination while having a good circulation on the portion of your body that you will apply it. This can help promote the growth of new hair.

One research found that peppermint oil, when utilized on mice, expanded the number of follicles for more opportunity of growing hair.

Blend 3 drops of peppermint basic oil with your preferred carrier oil. Backrub into your scalp, and let it sit for 5 minutes before washing out altogether with cleanser and conditioner.

Rosemary

If you need to improve both hair thickness and hair development, rosemary oil is a great choice because of its capacity to enhance our cells.

Blend a few drops of rosemary oil with olive or coconut oil, and apply it to your scalp. Let it sit for 10 minutes before washing it out with cleanser. Do this two times in seven days for more a desirable outcome.

Cedarwood

This essential oil is thought to promote hair development and diminish the usual male pattern baldness by adjusting the oil-producing organs in the scalp. It also has antifungal and antibacterial properties, which can treat various conditions that may add to dandruff or balding.

If you will put it into a blend with lavender, rosemary, and cedarwood it was found to diminish male pattern baldness in those with alopecia areata.

Blend a couple of drops of cedarwood essential oil with 1 tbsp of carrier oil of your preference. Backrub into your scalp, and abandon it on for 10 minutes before washing it out.

Lemongrass basic oil

Dandruff can be a big problem, and having a dandruff-free scalp is a significant piece of hair wellbeing. Lemongrass oil is a very effective dandruff treatment and it is better if you will add it to your daily regimen.

Blend a couple of drops into your shampoo and ensure it's rubbed really well into your scalp.

Chapter 6 – Essential Oil for Cancer and Other Diseases

I stand that one of the most useful types of herbal medicines in the world is essential oils. From triggering tranquility to calming our skin, aids healing and the combat certain illnesses, essential oils gives boundless opportunities to your well-being.

I'll just clarify that the utilization of these oils is not just a trend. Essential oils have been used already by our ancestors from the different portions of the world in ancient times.

Nowadays, my family and I utilized these oils in various uses in our everyday life. The purpose of these healing objects is pretty tremendous. I'll put a rundown of it, but some ways we usually utilize essential oils comprise as medicines, for hygiene, detoxification, and etc.

Why do we consider all of us must imitate us in utilizing essential oils as a basic necessity.

It's basic. We chose to utilize nonhazardous natural ways that have proven credibility in terms of their advantages, over a complete reliance on the prescribed medicines that are known for their side-effects.

Similarly, we opt to utilize own hygienic items and cleansers that are a great option because you are getting the cleansing power without the harmful chemicals. We get similar or even better outcomes while diminishing the hazards in our very own health.

I often questioned about the essential oils we prefer using to improve our overall health and prevent the formation of cancers, and also how we utilize them. This is the primary reason why I will share it to you so that you can also improve your health just like me and my family with the use of these essential oils.

Frankincense

Frankincense likely could be my absolute favorite essential oil because it fights certain tumors. It is mitigating, for one, which is imperative in the journey to recuperate from a lot of illnesses not only cancer. In particular, frankincense has been appeared to be an intense inhibitor of 5-lipoxygenase, a catalyst in charge of the immune system in the body.

It also helps support resistant capacity and anticipates sickness by duplicating white platelets and balancing invulnerable responses. It additionally improves flow, and decrease the pressure in our body. Oil of frankincense has appeared to contract and tone tissues, which speeds recovery.

Frankincense also appeared to give neurological help, including the capacity to get rid of poisons that may prompt neurological harm.

Nonetheless, it has a few advantages with regards to malignant tumor treatments, including relieving joint inflammation, equalizing hormones, empowering skin wellbeing, and helping assimilation.

Lavender

It has the phytochemicals perillyl liquor and linalool that are proven to drive malignant tumors away from our body.

It minimizes stress and supports the capacity of the immune system to perform better. Sleeping patterns are also improved with the use of this oil. Sadness and nervousness are completely taken away from our senses too. These go towards supporting the immune system in the battling of different illnesses.

Medical research has concluded that lavender essential oil is great in fighting different kinds of bacteria making the people who are using it really healthy.

Myrrh

Myrrh is considered as a very useful essential oil in the world of herbal medicines because it has a lot of incredible healing properties that. As far as disease healing is concerned, myrrh essential oil shows outstanding results in fighting malignant tumors.

It is also known to provide equilibrium in the hormones inside our body, which can be very crucial in healing. Like lavender and frankincense, It is also been utilized as a stress reliever.

Peppermint

It is a miracle oil with a wide scope of advantages. This essential oil's advantages in fighting cancers originate from its phytochemicals limonene, phytochemicals beta-caryophyllene, and beta-pinene, which are known for their effective detoxification properties.

Research says that this essential oil has the capacity to provide cell reinforcement and cancer-fighting agent properties which mostly concentrates on the prevention of tumor growth. It also contains antiangiogenic properties, which keep tumors from building up their own blood supply.

It also has antibacterial properties that make it really advantageous for fighting respiratory infection.

Turmeric

This essential oil has shown that if it is in a concentrated form, is known to battle malignant cells while advancing apoptosis resulting in a cancer-free body.

This very efficient essential oil has different advantages also that includes controlling glucose, help wounds heal rapidly, avert Alzheimer's illness, support you in getting a fit body, and simplicity joint pain.

How to Use Essential Oils for Healing?

Essential oils are so indispensable to my family's life, it's difficult to list each way we are using them! Whatever it may be, here are some top tips for utilizing essential oils in your everyday life.

- Put a drop behind your ears

  On a daily basis, I put myrrh and frankincense behind my ears and on the lymph hubs as a prophylactic (precaution insurance). Lavender or peppermint would be useful for respiratory issues, or basically to unwind. You can rub on the back of the skull, the bosoms, or the bottoms of your feet.

- Use a cool diffuser

  We want to diffuse essential oils all through our home. We do it for included mental lucidity. My office is constantly loaded up with the restorative smells of an assortment of essential oils.

- Massage into the skin

Some basic oils, similar to peppermint and clove, are exceptionally solid and it will become perfect if you will combine it with other types of oil

- You can utilize a decent quality, natural (ideally cool squeezed) oil like coconut, olive, or jojoba to blend in a couple of drops of your preferred fundamental oil.

  You would then be able to knead this straightforward "body margarine" onto your skin. For somewhat fancier body margarine, utilize a blender to whip strong coconut oil with fundamental oil. Utilize this blend to apply straightforwardly to influenced zones, (for example, with agony, joint pain, or stomach related problems), and for a snappy mind and other medical advantages.

- Ingest Internally

  One of my top pick, because I usually combine essential oils with my soothing beverages what I usually make is a so-called "Peppermint Lemonade."

I basically take 5-10 drops of peppermint essential oil, around twelve drops of lemon (or orange or tangerine oils, contingent upon my temperament), include water, some natural green stevia, and ice in an expansive pitcher. It's a super-quick, solid refreshment that I cherish. It's likewise delectable as a hot drink (utilize hot water and exclude the ice). In case you're simply making one glass at any given moment, utilize just 1 drop of peppermint + 1 drop of citrus oil. You can likewise utilize a couple of drops of essential oils in an unfilled gel container and swallow it.

- Toothpaste

You can make an assortment of individual items utilizing natural essential oils and other non-poisonous substances such as creams, face washes, mouthwash, cleansers. A toothpaste is anything but difficult to make but it proved me wrong because with the use of natural frankincense, myrrh, and coconut oil it became as easy as 1, 2, and 3.

Conclusion

That was a long ride, I hope that you have learned a lot from the essential oil recipes that we have tackled a while ago. Just one piece of advice before we part ways, I suggest that you must be creative when it comes to blending the various essential oils. The primary reason for this is that the recipes of essential oil blends are not just limited to the ones that are listed here because you can actually make one of your own depends on your needs.

Just make sure to study the different oils that are in this book so that the next time you plan to make your own recipe you will know the use of each essential oil which will help you make a very astounding recipe in the future.

But before anything else I would like to discuss to you the key points that you should remember if you want to use essential oils.

Quality

This is important to the point that it bears rehashing. Continuously utilize a top-quality, therapeutic essential oil. It ought to be ensured natural, and 100% unadulterated. Check the notoriety of your provider, and guarantee there are no fillers or added substances.

Keep oils from delicate territories

Essential oils are nature's powerhouses. Remember they are 40-50 times stronger than the plant itself. A few oils are progressively "fiery" than others. Some taste superior to other people.

Oregano is one that can consume a bit when you ingest it legitimately. Peppermint requires alert, and generally does best with a transporter oil when applying to the skin.

Never apply essential oils to touchy territories of the body, including the private areas or close to your eyes.

You ought to likewise test new oils to guarantee there are no responses before applying too generously.

You can begin by completing a sniff trial of the oil in the jug. In an instance that appears to be fine, at that point apply a spot of oil to within your wrist or arm, include a drop of oil and hold on to check whether there is any redness, tingling, or swelling.

Everyone's body is unique so you may need to attempt various oils to see which ones feel best to you.

Do not heat up oils

You've most likely observed or even have one of those oil burners for utilizing essential oils. What you can be sure of is that warming these oils decimates their healing properties. It's in every case best to utilize a cool diffuser. These are abundant and monetarily evaluated on the web.

Keep out of Children

Continuously be mindful when utilizing essential oils with kids. Dispersion is the most secure. For direct application, it's critical to weakening the more grounded oils, particularly with a decent oil. When making body spreads or back rub oils for kids, utilize 1 drop of essential oil to 4 tablespoons of other oils.

This will weaken the essential oil enough to make it progressively in the middle of the road and more secure for your kid. Be mindful so as not to put close to the eyes and dependably complete an allergy test first.

One word is very important in creating your own essential oil recipe which is "creativity" always apply that when you plan to make a recipe. So that's it I wish you good luck to your future endeavors.